20+ VEGAN DELICIOUS RECIPES

Mason Molina

Contents

Chapter One

INTRODUCTION

Followers of a vegan diet that excludes any animal-derived components are embracing a philosophy and way of life that can be pursued for a variety of reasons. The following is a succinct description of the primary causes.

Increasing your health's performance

Following the recommendations of the American Academy of Nutrition and Dietetics, well-planned vegetarian diets — including completely vegetarian or vegan diets — are healthy and nutritionally adequate, and they can give health benefits in the prevention and treatment of certain diseases. Vegetarian diets that are well-planned are appropriate for every stage of life, including pregnancy, lactation, infancy, youth, adolescence, and even for athletes, according to the American Dietetic Association.

Without a question, vegan food is among the healthiest foods available, and it has been shown to significantly reduce the incidence of illnesses and health conditions. For starters, vegans have significantly lower cholesterol levels than meat-eaters, and as a result, they are less likely to suffer from cardiovascular diseases than people who consume meat. To the extent that animal protein can be substituted for vegetable protein, it has been demonstrated that this can assist in lowering the level of cholesterol in the blood. Recent research has also revealed that a diet high in complex carbohydrates (which can only be obtained from plant foods) and low in fat is the most effective treatment for treating disorders such as diabetes. In contrast, vegetable fats have been shown to lower arterial pressure whereas animal fats have been shown to raise it.

Vegans are less likely than non-vegans to suffer from heart disease, as well as hypertension, obesity, diabetes, cancer, intestinal diseases, kidney and vesicle stones, and osteoporosis, to name a few illnesses.

Any doctor would recommend that you eat a diet that is low in fat and high in fiber and vitamins.

The World Health Organization (WHO) itself recommends that people reduce their intake of fats while increasing their intake of fruits, vegetables, grains, and legumes, which are all essential vegan food items. It is necessary for our bodies to be protected from external aggression that antioxidants such as those found in fruits and vegetables be consumed.

Carbohydrates, on the other hand, are one of the most essential sources of energy for the body, and the vegan diet is abundant in this element due to the richness of fruits, cereals, legumes, and vegetables. Finally, it is important to note that vegetables are the foods that have the highest concentrations of vitamins, minerals, and fiber.

Increasing the ease with which one digests

There are increasing numbers of people who suffer from dyspepsia on a regular basis, which is almost always the result of a nutrient-deficient diet. It is critical to consume a sufficient amount of fiber in order to avoid this. This aids in the flow of digested food through the small and large intestines, as well as the absorption of vitamins and minerals and the elimination of toxins from the body by the body. When it comes to maintaining proper digestive system function and avoiding problems such as being overweight or obese, a vegan diet is the best choice.

A vegan's grocery list, which contains all kinds of fruits, vegetables, cereals, and, in general, any other ingredients that are part of a vegan diet, is far less expensive than an omnivore's list, which includes meat, fish, shellfish, and dairy products, among other things. Nonetheless, if you want to minimize your expenditure even further, you might consider the following suggestions:

Make a plan for your meals. Spend 15 minutes once a week planning your food for the next 7 days and creating a shopping list with everything you'll need to prepare it (Sunday afternoon could be a good time to do this).

Put your faith in the foundational ingredients of your vegan diet. In general, they are less expensive, and their variety allows for an almost limitless number of different dishes to be created. For example, beans are inexpensive, long-lasting, and versatile, allowing for a variety of flavor combinations depending on how they are prepared and the items that are served with them.

Fruits and vegetables that are in season should be purchased. Whenever you go shopping, you will always be able to find seasonal products that are significantly less expensive and more delicious.

Make a large amount of food. Plan to prepare a significant quantity of a single dish once a week and then freeze it so that you can eat it over the course of several days. Prepare meals with components that may be rationed, such as cooked beans, spaghetti sauces, and vegetable stock, to save money.

Reduce your intake of protein to a reasonable level.

Protein is required for the growth and maintenance of all tissues and organs. There are a number of amino acids in it, all of which are important for the correct development of the human body. The majority of foods contain protein in some form, whether in minor or big quantities. High quality protein is defined as protein that contains all of the essential amino acids required by the organism. Some foods contain a higher concentration of necessary amino acids than others, but the key is knowing how to combine them so that the body receives an adequate supply of these important amino acids. Vegans who eat a well-balanced diet consisting of grains, legumes, seeds, nuts, and vegetables acquire their protein from a variety of sources that are good in quality.

Protein should account for around 15% of total calories in a well-balanced diet. However, most of the time, people consume an excess of 25% protein while consuming insufficient amounts of other vital nutrients like as carbs and fat. The vegan diet enables one to limit the intake of excessive calories.

A high protein diet can be harmful to one's health in the long run, according to some experts. An excessive protein consumption, on the other hand, has been shown to accelerate calcium loss from the body, resulting in the beginning of disorders such as osteoporosis and osteopenia.

Taking care of the environment

It has been determined by the United Nations Food and Agriculture Organization (FAO) that the livestock sector generates more greenhouse gases than the transportation sector. As a result, it is one of the most significant factors contributing to the degradation of groundwater and hydrological resources. In one of their latest publications, the Food and Agriculture Organization of the United Nations said unequivocally:

It is anticipated that agricultural impacts will expand significantly as a result of population growth, which will result in increased consumption of animal products. In contrast to fossil fuels, it is difficult to find alternatives because people need to eat. A significant reduction in these consequences can only be achieved with a significant shift in the global population's dietary patterns, which includes a significant shift away from animal-based products.

We can all agree that lowering, if not fully eliminating, our intake of meat and its derivatives is a positive step toward lessening our environmental impact on the earth.

Three sauces on tubers

45 minutes for 6 persons Difficulty\sIngredients

a couple of parsnips

2 Yukon Gold or golden potatoes, preferably

two beets

1 pound of sweet potato

1 garlic clove

3 tblsp. extra virgin olive oil

salt (two tablespoons)

a pinch of ground black pepper

Dressing for Caesar salad

To make the aioli, combine the following ingredients in a mixing bowl.

12 cup soy milk, 125 mL

Sunflower oil, 250 mL (12 cup)

1 teaspoon sodium chloride

two garlic cloves

a single lemon

To make the wild sauce, combine the following ingredients.

Aioli, 180 mL (34 cup)

1 tablespoon paprika (smoked)

1 Place all of the tubers in a baking dish, peeled and cubed.

2 Halve the garlic head and place it in the baking dish.

3 Combine the oil, salt, and pepper in a mixing bowl. Mix thoroughly.

4 Cover the dish with aluminum foil and bake for 25 minutes at 180°C (350°F).

minutes.

5 Blend the soy milk, sunflower oil, and salt together in an electric blender until a mayonnaise develops.

6 Toss in the lemon and garlic cloves. Continue emulsifying until the aioli is smooth and homogeneous.

7 Mix in the smoked paprika with the aioli.

8 Arrange the tubers on a serving platter with the Caesar dressing, aioli, and wild sauce.

The Yukon Gold potato is ideal for frying or baking. They're noted for their silky smoothness.

Chapter Two

SEITAN,ROASTED POTATOES AND MORE

Creamed seitan, roasted sweet potato, and onion caramelized

30 minutes for 6 persons Difficulty

Ingredients

Olive oil is a type of oil that comes from

12 fillets de seitan

2 packets cream cheese spread (vegetarian)

seasoning with salt and pepper

3 steamed sweet potatoes

3 onions (red)

Sugar

1 Lightly brown the seitan on a grill pan with a little oil.

2 Add the cream and a bit of salt and pepper to taste. Cook for another couple of minutes over medium heat.

3 Wrap the sweet potatoes individually in aluminum foil and bake for 20 minutes or until soft in an oven preheated to 180°C (350°F).

4 Cut the onions into slices and sauté them with a little sugar in a covered pot over low heat until they start to caramelize.

5 Slice the sweet potato and serve it alongside the caramelized onion and the creamed seitan.

Seitan is high in protein, but it's also low in calories, lowers cholesterol, and has far more calcium and micronutrients than meat.

If you'd rather...

You can also use small chunks of butternut squash instead of sweet potatoes, which you will roast in the oven.

Chapter Three

SEITAN PICCATA

Piccata de seitan con creme de spinach

40 minutes x 6 people

Ingredients

For the spinach, follow these instructions:

12 smoked tofu block

12 oz. tofu (natural)

2 tbsp yeast (brewer's yeast)

two garlic cloves

a single onion

Mushrooms, 250 g (12 lb)

1 spinach bag (frozen)

Vegetable broth, 400 mL (about 1 and 34 cups)

Oil

To make the sauce, combine the following ingredients.

Oil

6 cloves of garlic

1 glass white wine

12 liters (2 cups) vegetable broth

lemons (two)

12 tblsp capers (or 3 large caper-berries)

2 tbsp yeast (brewer's yeast)

1 tablespoon cornmeal (corn flour preferred)

Salt

For the fillets, prepare as follows:

12 fillets de seitan

2 cups flour (whole wheat)

1 CUP BAKED BAKED BAKED BAKED BAKED B

1 tblsp. fresh thyme

1 tblsp oregano (oregano)

salt (1 tablespoon)

1 teaspoon of black pepper

mustard (1 tablespoon)

1 In a mixing dish, combine both varieties of tofu and the brewer's yeast for the spinach.

Add water in small increments until the texture is smooth and creamy.

2 Sweat the garlic and chopped onion in a pan with a tablespoon of oil. Add the sliced mushrooms when they begin to brown.

3 Allow the spinach and 250 mL (1 cup) of vegetable broth to reduce until there is hardly no liquid remaining. Add the tofu cream and simmer for 3 minutes over very low heat, covered tightly. Set aside after seasoning with salt and pepper.

4 It's time to start making the sauce. Sweat the peeled and sliced garlic in a pan with 1 tablespoon of oil. Pour in the wine and reduce it by half. 150 mL (about 23 cups) vegetable broth, lemon juice, capers, brewer's yeast, maize flour (dissolved in a little amount of water), and salt Allow time for this to cook.

5 Combine the whole-wheat flour, bread crumbs, herbs, and a pinch of salt in a mixing bowl. In a separate dish, whisk together the mustard and 4 cups of water until no lumps remain.

6 Dredge the seitan in the flour mixture first, then in the mustard, using two forks.

Repeat this step a few times more, and then fry the seitan in batches in a hot pan. Drain the seitan by placing it on top of an absorbent paper towel.

7 Place the creamy spinach, 2 seitan fillets, and piccata sauce on top of each dish. Serve with lemon slices as a garnish.

A clever ruse

Use capers cured in dry salt, which are commonly used in Italian cuisine, to make this meal even more delicious.

Seitan slices in a mushroom sauce, and

mille-feuille de pommes

50 minutes x 6 people x 6 people x 6 people x 6 people x 6 people Difficulty

Ingredients

For mille-feuille, use the following formula:

Potatoes, 500 g (1 lb)

2 shallots

4 garlic cloves, bay leaves, thyme, salt, pepper, and olive oil To make the sauce, combine the following ingredients.

12 garlic bulb

2 onions, chopped

extra virgin olive oil

2 quarts red wine

12 pound of common mushrooms (250 g)

shiitake mushrooms, 250 g (12 lb)

1 toasted slice of bread

1 quart vegetable stock

brewer's yeast (2 tablespoons), sage, basil, salt, and pepper
For the fillets, prepare as follows:

12 fillets de seitan

flour (two cups)

1 CUP BAKED BAKED BAKED BAKED BAKED B

1 tblsp. fresh thyme

1 tblsp oregano (oregano)

salt (1 tablespoon)

1 teaspoon of black pepper

paprika (2 tablespoons)

four cups of water

a quarter-cup of soy sauce

1 Make the mille-feuille first. Cut the potatoes and onions into pieces to begin. Cut the garlic cloves into little pieces after that.

Mix them with the herbs (to taste), olive oil, and a bit of salt and pepper in a large mixing basin.

2 Place the mixture in an aluminum foil-lined baking dish and bake at 180°C for 30 minutes.

(350°F) until the potatoes are fork-tender.

3 Carry on with the sauce now. With a skillet, brown the garlic and chopped onion.

a dash of olive oil Add the wine and reduce to roughly   of its volume.

4 Cook for about 20 minutes over low heat in a covered saucepan with the common mushrooms, shiitakes, and toasted bread.

5 Cook for 15 minutes after adding the veggie broth. Season with salt and pepper after adding the herbs to taste.

6 Combine the flour, bread crumbs, herbs, paprika, and a pinch of salt in a mixing bowl. Mix the 4 cups of water with a little soy sauce in a separate basin to give it color.

7 Dredge the seitan in flour first, then in soy sauce, using a pair of forks.

This process should be repeated twice more. In a skillet with plenty of oil, fry the seitan in batches and drain on paper towels.

8 Arrange some of the sauce, a piece of mille-feuille, and the seitan fillets on a serving platter.

Shiitake mushrooms are high in fiber, low in calories, and provide the majority of essential amino acids.

They're ideal for creating broth or including into stews.

Chapter Four

SHISH KEBAB

with seitan

20 minutes x 6 people x 6 people x 6 people x 6 people x 6 persons Difficulty

Ingredients

Seitan chunks (60 oz) (evenly cut)

Olive oil is a type of oil that comes from

seasoning with salt and pepper

Skewers are a type of skewer (metal or wooden)

For the marinade, combine the following ingredients.

parsley, 1 bunch

a single onion

three garlic cloves

paprika, 3 teaspoons

Salt

1 cup extra virgin olive oil

1 Chop the parsley, onion, and garlic finely and combine with the paprika, salt, and olive oil in a mixing bowl.

2 Thread the seitan onto the skewers (2 skewers per dinner guest) and marinate them overnight.

3 Heat the oil in a pan the next day and sear the skewers over medium heat.

Serve immediately, with bread on the side.

A clever ruse

It's better to marinate the skewers overnight to make them more delicious.

Chapter Five

GNOCCHI

Gnocchi with a sauce of pepper, walnuts, and basil

45 minutes for 6 persons Difficulty

Ingredients

2 packages gnocchi (fresh gnocchi best)

2 courgettes

To make the sauce, combine the following ingredients.

3 peppers (red)

three garlic cloves

200 g (7 oz) walnuts—approximately 12 cup

basil, 1 bunch

12 cup extra virgin olive oil

seasoning with salt and pepper

1 Begin by preparing the sauce. In a baking dish, combine the peppers and garlic; cover with aluminum foil and bake at 180°C (350°F) until the peppers are nicely roasted.

2 Spread the walnuts on a separate pan and toast them in the oven until they are nicely toasted.

3 Peel the peppers and garlic and combine them with the walnuts, basil, oil, salt, and pepper in a blender. Blend until the sauce is smooth and homogeneous.

4 Zucchini should be cut into small, homogeneous cubes. Then, with a little oil, salt, and pepper, sauté them.

5 Cook the gnocchi and serve with 1 tablespoon of pepper sauce and a few zucchini slices.

Chapter Six

PENNE PASTA

Penne with olives, spinach, and garlic oil

asparagus

15 minutes for 6 persons Difficulty

Ingredients

12 cup almonds, sliced

1 cup extra virgin olive oil

3 asparagus bunches

garlic cloves (eight)

12 cup extra virgin olive oil

a handful of spinach

Penne pasta, 600 g (21 oz)

1 Preheat the oven to 350°F and roast the almonds until golden brown.

2 Prepare the olives by pitting and slicing them.

3 Cut the asparagus into crosswise strips, blanch for 1 minute, then shock in cold water immediately.

4 Chop the garlic cloves finely.

5 In a skillet, heat the olive oil and sauté the asparagus and garlic until well browned. Remove the pan from the heat and stir in the spinach, olives, and almonds.

6 Cook the pasta and toss it with the sauce you just prepared.

A clever ruse

You can add a pinch of chili pepper to the flavor to make it more intense and spicy.

Leeks, dried tomatoes, and basil sauce on tagliatelle.

25 minutes x 6 people x 6 people x 6 people x 6 people x 6 people Difficulty

Ingredients

Olive oil is a type of oil that comes from

seasoning with salt and pepper

12 oz. white wine

5 sliced leeks

2 tomatoes (dried)

5 leaves of basil

Pine nuts, 200 g (7 oz)

Tagliatelle pasta, 660 g (about 23 oz)

1 Braise the sliced leeks in a pot with a little oil, a touch of salt, pepper, and the wine until they are lovely and soft.

2 Blend the ingredients, along with the dried tomatoes and basil, in a blender.

Add a little water until it reaches a creamy consistency.

3 Toast the pine nuts in the oven and then toss them whole into the leek sauce.

4 Cook the pasta until al dente, then drain and toss with the sauce.

A clever ruse

Before serving, add extra spices to the meal to enhance the flavor.

Chapter Seven

LINGUINE

Butternut squash and caper linguine

30 minutes for 6 persons Difficulty

Ingredients

1 butternut squash, big

Olive oil is a type of oil that comes from

a single onion

three garlic cloves

1 bottle of beer, preferably dark

seasoning with salt and pepper

12 tblsp capers (or 3 large caper-berries)

linguine, 900 g (2 lbs)

1 Prepare the butternut squash by peeling and dicing it.

2 Sweat the onions and thinly sliced garlic in a pot with heated oil until they are transparent. Combine the chopped butternut squash, dark beer, salt, and pepper in a mixing bowl.

Cover the pot and cook on low heat until the butternut squash is soft, about 30 minutes.

3 Add the capers to the pot after washing them to remove any extra salt. Keep the pot covered over the heat for another minute, then blend until the sauce is smooth and homogeneous. Salt & pepper to taste.

4 Boil the linguine and toss with the butternut squash and caper sauce before serving.

Linguine is a sort of pasta that originated in Campania, Italy, and is extremely similar to spaghetti. Because of its form, this pasta works well with a variety of sauces and sides.

Chapter Eight

RISOTTO WITH MUSHROOMS AND ARTICHOKES

20 minutes x 6 people

Ingredients

2 shallots

two garlic cloves

Olive oil is a type of oil that comes from

1 bottle of beer, preferably dark

300 g (10.5 oz) brown rice (about 12 cups)

2 artichoke hearts

250 g (12 pound) shiitake mushrooms

seasoning with salt and pepper

Broth made from vegetables

1 The onion and garlic should be peeled and sliced into very small chunks, then sautéed in a little olive oil. Continue to heat

until the beer has completely reduced. Combine the rice and the other ingredients.

2 Chop the artichokes and garlic cloves. Sauté and brown the vegetables in a pan with oil.

3 Slice the mushrooms and sauté them in a little oil and salt until they're well browned. Remove the pan from the heat and combine the mushrooms and artichokes in a separate bowl. Remove from the equation.

4 Boil the rice in a pot with some of the broth until the liquid has reduced by about half. Add a large handful of the mushroom and artichoke combination right away.

5 Season to taste with salt and pepper before serving.

Chapter Nine

YAKITORI

yakitori, rice sautéed with napa cabbage

carrots roasted with mint tofu

40 minutes x 6 people

Ingredients

12 a head of napa cabbage

1 teaspoon sodium chloride

Pepper

Olive oil is a type of oil that comes from

300 g (10.5 oz) brown rice (about 12 cup)

1 glass red wine

a quarter cup of soy sauce

12 cup sugar

1 pound of tofu

Carrots (five)

mint leaves, 1 bundle

sunflower oil (14 cup)

2 tblsp sesame seed oil

chopped fresh spinach

1 Slice the napa cabbage and sauté it with a little salt, pepper, and olive oil until soft. Combine the rice and the other ingredients.

2 To make the yakitori, whisk together the wine, soy sauce, and sugar in a mixing dish until the sugar is completely dissolved.

3 Slice the tofu and lay it in a baking dish with a little oil and the yakitori on top. Bake for 15 minutes at 180°C (350°F) or until the tofu is well browned.

4 Carrots should be peeled and chopped lengthwise.

5 Combine the mint, sunflower oil, sesame oil, and salt in a blender until no lumps remain.

6 In a baking tray, combine the carrots and the mint oil and bake at 180°C (350°F) until the carrots are soft.

7 Arrange the rice on a plate with the tofu, carrots, and chopped spinach.

Chapter Ten

FRESH RISOTTO

Rice with butternut squash cooked in thyme,

sautéed walnuts and a leek sauce

30 minutes for 6 persons Difficulty

Ingredients

1 butternut squash, big

Thyme

two garlic cloves

300 g (10.5 oz) walnuts (about 12 cups)

3 tblsp. extra virgin olive oil

a third of a cup of soy sauce

300 g (10.5 oz) boiling brown rice (about 12 cups)

To make the sauce, combine the following ingredients.

four leeks

seasoning with salt and pepper

a bottle of white wine (about 12 oz.)

Olive oil is a type of oil that comes from

Milk made from soy beans

Nutmeg

1 Heat the olive oil in a pot, then add the sliced leeks, a pinch of salt, a pinch of pepper, and the wine. Continue to cook until all of the alcohol has been removed.

2 In a blender or thermomix, combine the ingredients and add a splash of soy milk and grated nutmeg for a creamier texture.

3 Butternut squash should be peeled and diced. Place the butternut squash chunks in a baking tray with the thyme and garlic cloves, cover with aluminum foil, and bake at 180°C (350°F) until soft.

4 With the oil and soy sauce, sauté the walnuts until they begin to brown.

5 Put some walnuts in a bowl to use as a mold, then a layer of butternut squash, then the brown rice on top. Turn it over onto a platter, pressing down firmly but gently to keep the shape. Serve with the sauce.

Chapter Eleven

TOFU

Tofu in a sweet and sour sauce, as well as

sesame-oil-dressed veggies

20 minutes x 6 people

Ingredients

12 fillets of tofu

Flour

1 asparagus bushel

1 broccoli floret

Sesame seed oil

2 peppers (red)

1 onion, red

2 carrots, peeled

seasoning with salt and pepper

To make the sauce, combine the following ingredients.

a quarter of a pineapple, diced

1 quart vegetable stock

12 cup sugar

a quarter cup of apple cider

vinegar

14 cup ketchup

corn starch, 1 teaspoon

seasoning with salt and pepper

1 Make the sweet and sour sauce first. To do so, combine all of the ingredients in a pot (excluding the cornstarch) and boil over low heat until the vinegar has entirely evaporated. To keep the sauce from sticking to the bottom of the saucepan, dissolve the cornstarch in a little water, then add it to the pot and stir well.

2 With a shallow dish, dredge the tofu fillets in flour. Then, in a large skillet with plenty of oil, brown the tofu on all sides.

3 Blanch the asparagus and broccoli in boiling water for 1 minute, then shock them in cold water.

4 Heat the sesame oil in a skillet and add the peppers, onion, broccoli, asparagus, and carrots to cook. Salt & pepper to taste.

5 Finally, arrange the sautéed veggies alongside the tofu fillets and sweet and sour sauce on a serving platter.

» Tofu is an unrivaled source of high-quality vegetable protein that may be fried, battered, stewed, grilled, and even used in soups, sauces, and desserts.

« Sesame oil has a pleasant flavor and scent. It's crucial that it's unrefined because it'll keep all of its nutritional benefits (rich in iron, magnesium, and vitamin E).

Chapter Twelve

PATE'

rosemary, red pepper, and macadamia nut pâté

35 minutes for 6 people Difficulty

Ingredients

5 peppers (red)

200 g (7 oz) macadamia nuts (about 1 cup)

4 sprigs rosemary

8 tblsp. extra virgin olive oil

a grain of salt

a pinch of salt

1 Char the peppers whole in the oven for 20 minutes at 180°C (350°F).

minutes. Allow them to cool to room temperature after that.

2 Preheat the oven to 180°C (350°F) and roast the walnuts for 3 minutes.

3 Peel the peppers and combine them with the walnuts, rosemary, oil, and a touch of salt and pepper in a blender. Blend until the mixture is smooth and homogeneous in consistency.

4 Serve the pâté with raw vegetables or rye bread as a side dish.

Macadamia nuts, sometimes known as Queensland nuts, are prized for their delicate flavor and silky texture. They're high in calories (about 700 calories per 100 g, or 3.5 oz) and high in protein, carbs, and fiber.

Chapter Thirteen

PAELLA WITH MUSHROOMS AND ROSEMARY

45 minutes for 6 persons Difficulty

Ingredients

a single onion

two garlic cloves

3 tblsp. extra virgin olive oil

2 tomatoes, red

Common mushrooms, 100 g (3.5 oz)

Oyster mushrooms, 100 g (3.5 oz)

rice (six cups)

four saffron strands

Peas, 50 g (a bit less than 2 oz)

a grain of salt

a pinch of salt

1 rosemary sprig 1 rosemary sprig 1 rosemary sprig 1 rosemary

Broth made from vegetables

Green onion or parsley

1 Peel the onion and garlic and cut them into very small pieces.

2 In a paella pan, heat the oil and add the garlic and onion. Cook for 2 minutes over medium heat.

3 Cube the tomatoes and toss them into the paella.

4 Both varieties of mushrooms should be sliced. Cook for 3 minutes after adding the mushrooms to the paella.

minutes.

5 Combine the rice, saffron, peas, salt, pepper, and rosemary in a mixing bowl.

6 Cover the rice with vegetable stock and simmer over low heat, stirring occasionally, until it is done.

7 Garnish with parsley leaves or green onions before serving.

10 Add the red wine, smashed tomatoes, sliced carrots, salt, and pepper to the pan.

Cook, stirring occasionally, until the wine has reduced by half.

11 Stir in the vegetable broth well.

12 Arrange the meatballs in a baking dish and cover with the wine braising liquid. Add a few cilantro leaves as a finishing touch.

Chapter Fourteen

PASTA WITH GREEN PEPPER

6 participants 25 minutes Difficulty

Ingredients

two seitan packages

2 peppers, green

3 tblsp. extra virgin olive oil

Soy veggie cream cheese, 500 mL (2 cups)

salt (1 tablespoon)

1 teaspoon cayenne

Spaghetti, 600 g (21 oz)

1 Set aside the seitan and peppers, which should be cut into large cubes.

2 In a medium-sized pan, heat the oil and cook the peppers for a few minutes.

3 Add the seitan and stir thoroughly for 5 minutes, making sure nothing sticks.

4 Combine the cream, salt, and pepper in a mixing bowl. Cook for another 2 minutes on low heat.

5 Boil the spaghetti until it is al dente in a big pot.

6 To serve, spoon a piece of the pasta onto a plate and top with the seitan sauce.

7 Add salt and pepper to taste.

Seitan is highly suggested for athletes or people who are physically active due to its high protein content. It's also good for pregnant women, newborns, adolescents, and convalescents.

Chapter Fifteen

POLENTA WITH MUSHROOMS

50 minutes 6 persons Difficulty

Ingredients

1 quart (about 1 liter) of water

a single garlic bulb

1 cauliflower

a single onion

1 stalk celery

rosemary, chopped

a grain of salt

a pinch of salt

Instant polenta (200 g/7 oz)

18 fresh mushrooms (about 1 pound; oyster mushrooms best)

Olive oil is a type of oil that comes from

Aioli (250 mL/1 cup)

1 tablespoon marcona almonds (preferably peeled)

Sauces from Italy, such as Romesco

1 Boil the garlic, carrot, onion, and celery for 10 minutes in a pot of boiling water.

2 Strain the broth and season with a teaspoon of salt and pepper and half of the chopped rosemary.

3 Bring the broth to a boil with the instant polenta (following the package instructions).

4 In a flat baking dish, spread the polenta.

5 Let it rest for 30 minutes before using a cookie cutter to cut out multiple circles.

6 Arrange 18 polenta rounds in a baking tray and top each with an oyster mushroom.

7 Drizzle a little oil over each slice and season with salt, pepper, and chopped rosemary with a basting brush.

8 Preheat oven to 200°C (400°F) and bake for 10 minutes.

9 In a blender, combine the aioli and almonds and emulsify them.

10 For each guest, serve 3 slices of polenta with Romesco sauce and almond aioli.

Chapter Sixteen

FEIJOADA

35 minutes 6 persons Difficulty

Ingredients

two garlic cloves

3 tblsp. extra virgin olive oil

1 cauliflower

1 courgette

a single eggplant

1 pound of seitan

500 g (about 1 pound) cooked black beans

Vegetable broth, 250 mL (1 cup)

1 smoked tofu packet

salt (1 tablespoon)

1 teaspoon cayenne

10 leaves of parsley

1 Peel and thinly slice the garlic cloves.

2 Lightly sauté the garlic in a skillet with oil.

3 Prepare the carrots by peeling and dicing them. Cook for 3 minutes after adding them to the pan.

4 Toss in the zucchini, eggplant, and seitan, which has been chopped into large cubes. Cook for another 10 minutes on low heat with the pan covered.

5 Combine the beans and vegetable broth in a large mixing bowl. Over medium heat, cook for 5 minutes.

6 Add the tofu to the pan, cut into large cubes. Remove the pan from the heat, season with salt and pepper, and stir well.

7 Garnish with parsley leaves and serve the feijoada.

Feijoada is a meal that is synonymous with Brazilian and Portuguese cuisine.

Because this meal is heavy in calories, it's better to limit yourself to just one serving, ideally during the cooler months.

Chapter Seventeen

PEPPERS WITH QUINOA

6 participants 40 minutes Difficulty

Ingredients

6 peppers, red

a head of cauliflower (12 oz.)

a head of broccoli (12 oz.)

3 green garlic stalks

1 quart (1.1 liters) of water

quinoa (3 cups)

Parsley

Toasted almonds, 100 g (3.5 oz)

1 pound of tofu

To make the sauce, combine the following ingredients.

two garlic cloves

cumin, a pinch

2 tablespoons of vegetable oil

three carrots

Vegetable broth, 250 mL (1 cup)

a grain of salt

a pinch of salt

1 Preheat the oven to 180°C (350°F) and bake the peppers for 20 minutes. Remove the skin and stems after they have cooled.

2 Chop the broccoli and cauliflower into small pieces.

3 Cook the broccoli for 2 minutes on high heat. Remove the pieces from the water, drain carefully, and place them in cold water.

4 Cook the cauliflower for 4 minutes in the same water. Drain the water thoroughly and rinse the pieces in cold water.

5 Sauté the sliced green garlic, broccoli, and cauliflower in a skillet with a little oil, salt, and pepper.

6 Bring the water (1.1 l, or slightly over 1 quart) to a boil in a saucepan with a pinch of salt.

When the water begins to boil, add the quinoa and cook for 12 minutes over low heat, covered.

7 Chop the parsley and almonds into small pieces. Combine the quinoa and the sauce.

8 Toss the tofu with the quinoa and cut it into strips.

9 Using a baking ring, place the quinoa in the bottom of a dish and top with the sautéed broccoli and cauliflower.

10 In a skillet with oil, saute the sliced garlic and cumin to prepare the sauce. Add the carrots to the pan after peeling and slicing them into thin half-moon shapes. Add the veggie broth, salt, and pepper to taste. Over medium heat, cook for 10 minutes. Using an electric blender, combine the ingredients together.

11 Toss the quinoa mixture and vegetables into each pepper. Serve with carrot sauce on the side.

Pie with mushrooms and peas

6 participants 25 minutes Difficulty

Ingredients

To make the dough, combine the flour, baking powder, and salt.

Wheat flour, 400 g (14 oz)

margarine, 200 g (7 oz)

3 tblsp. ice-cold water

For the filling, combine:

3 tblsp. extra virgin olive oil

two garlic cloves

2 shallots

Mushrooms, 200 g (7 oz)

2 tablespoons bourbon

100 g (3.5 oz) peas (about 12 cup)

1 teaspoon sodium chloride

1 teaspoon cayenne

6 leaves of parsley

80 g (3 oz) cornstarch—approximately 14 cup

80 g (3 fl oz) water—approximately 13 cup

1 In a mixing basin, combine all of the dough ingredients until they create a homogenous dough. Wrap in plastic wrap and place in the refrigerator while you prepare the stew.

2 Fry the peeled and sliced garlic for 2 minutes in a pan with oil.

3 Toss the onions, peeled and chopped, into the pan. 4 minutes in the oven

4 Add the brandy and the cut mushrooms. Cook for 5 minutes over medium heat.

minutes, stirring constantly to avoid the mixture sticking together.

5 Toss in the peas, salt, pepper, and parsley leaves in the end. Remove the pan from the heat and stir thoroughly.

6 Combine the cornstarch and water in a bowl and stir into the stew.

7 Place the dough in a round shape and roll it out. Prick the bottom with a fork and place the stew in the center.

8 To prevent the dough from blowing out during the baking process, cover with extra dough and prick it again.

9 Drizzle a little olive oil over the top and bake at 180°C (350°F) until beautifully browned.

Chapter Eighteen

PIZZA WITH BASIL AND ARTICHOKES

50 minutes 6 persons Difficulty

Ingredients

To make the dough, combine the flour, baking powder, and salt.

150 g (5.3 oz) wheat flour—approximately 12 cup

100 g (3.5 fl oz) water—approximately 12 cup

1 teaspoon sodium chloride

sugar (one teaspoon)

12 ounces (15 g) fresh yeast

1 tablespoon extra virgin olive oil

To make the icing:

4 tbsp. crushed tomatoes

4 tomatoes (fresh)

1 onion, green

12 oil on canvas artichokes

2 tblsp. extra virgin olive oil

a grain of salt

a pinch of salt

Leaves of basil

1 Combine the flour, water, salt, sugar, yeast, and olive oil in a mixing bowl.

2 On a hard surface, knead the dough thoroughly and let it rest for 20 minutes.

3 Sprinkle a little flour on the work surface and roll out the dough. Place it on a pizza pan and bake it.

4 Using a fork, prick the dough and cover with crushed tomatoes.

5 Preheat the oven to 180°C (355°F) and bake the dough for 5 minutes.

6 Take the dough out of the oven.

7 Slice the tomatoes thinly. The onion should be peeled and chopped into small strips. Artichokes should be cut in half.

8 Arrange tomato slices, onion slices, artichokes, olive oil, salt, and pepper on top of the pizza.

9 Bake for 15 minutes at 180°C (350°F). Serve the basil leaves on top of the pizza.

Chapter Nineteen

PIZZA WITH TOMATOES AND CHEESE

Pizza with sun-dried tomatoes and cashew cheese

30 minutes 6 people Difficulty

Ingredients

To make the dough, combine the flour, baking powder, and salt.

150 g (5.3 oz) wheat flour—approximately 12 cup

100 g (3.5 fl oz) water—approximately 12 cup

1 teaspoon sodium chloride

sugar (one teaspoon)

12 ounces (15 g) fresh yeast

1 tablespoon extra virgin olive oil

To make the cheese:

Cashews, 100 g (3.5 oz)

400 mL (about 14 fl oz) water

2 tbsp yeast (brewer's yeast)

1 teaspoon sodium chloride

4 tbsp. crushed tomatoes

To make the icing:

a total of 6 cherry tomatoes

12 Tomatoes, Dried

18 leaves of arugula

Leaves of oregano

1 Combine the flour, water, salt, sugar, yeast, and olive oil in a mixing bowl.

2 On a hard surface, knead the dough thoroughly and let it rest for 20 minutes.

3 Sprinkle a little flour on the work surface and roll out the dough. Place it on a pizza pan and bake it.

4 Using a fork, prick the dough and cover with crushed tomatoes.

5 Preheat the oven to 180°C (350°F) and bake the dough for 5 minutes.

6 Take the dough out of the oven.

7 To prepare the cheese, in an electric blender, combine the cashews, water, brewer's yeast, and salt until you have a smooth, lump-free sauce.

8 Halve the cherry tomatoes and thinly slice the dried tomatoes.

9 Arrange the cashew cheese, dried tomatoes, cherry tomatoes, and arugula on top of the pizza. Preheat oven to 180°C (350°F) and bake for 15 minutes.

10 Remove the pizza from the oven and garnish with oregano leaves.

Chapter Twenty

BROWNIES

1 hour 6 people Difficulty

Ingredients

300 g (10.5 oz) flour (about 2 58 cups)

1 teaspoon sodium chloride

350 g (approximately 12 oz) brown sugar

1 teaspoon powdered baking soda

1 oz. cocoa powder (30 g)

Semisweet chocolate, 200 g (7 oz)

margarine, 200 g (7 oz)

Water, 250 mL (9 fl oz)

1 teaspoon vanilla extract

walnuts, 50 g (approximately 2 oz)

1 Combine the flour, salt, sugar, baking powder, and cocoa powder in a mixing dish.

2 In a medium saucepan, melt the chocolate and margarine together.

3 Combine the flour, melted chocolate, water, vanilla, and walnuts in a mixing bowl.

4 Pour the batter into a 20 x 40 cm (8 x 16 in) baking sheet and bake for 50 minutes at 150°C (300°F).

5 Allow the brownies to cool completely before cutting them into little rectangles.

Brownies are a sort of chocolate cake popular in the United States that was produced as a result of a culinary mishap: it is reported that a North American cook was cooking a cake at the end of the nineteenth century and failed to include a leavening agent.

Chapter Twenty-one

CHOCOLATE COOKIES

30 minutes 6 people Difficulty

Ingredients

50 g (about 3 oz) candied oranges

flour, 300 g (10.5 oz)

1 teaspoon sodium chloride

brown sugar, 200 g (7 oz)

12 tsp. bicarbonate of soda

100 g (3.5 oz) chocolate chips (about 12 cup)

300 g (10.5 oz) margarine (approximately 2 12 sticks)

1 teaspoon vanilla extract

1 Using a knife, finely cut the candied oranges.

2 Combine the flour, salt, sugar, and baking soda in a mixing basin.

3 Combine the chocolate chips, margarine, and vanilla extract in a mixing bowl. Mix everything together until you have a solid dough.

4 Roll out a few cookies and lay them on a baking pan.

5 Bake the biscuits at 180°C (350°F) until golden brown around the edges. Allow to cool on a rack before serving.

Round cookies with chocolate chips are known as Chocolate Chip Cookies. There are endless varieties of this dish, which is popular in English-speaking countries.

If you'd rather...

1 orange, 250 g (8 oz) sugar, and 200 g (7 fl oz) water are required to produce candied oranges. Slice the oranges and cook them for about 2 hours over low heat with the sugar and water.

Chapter Twenty-two

CHOCOLATE AND BANANAS MUFFINS

30 minutes 6 people Difficulty

Ingredients

310 g (11 oz) flour (about 2 34 cups)

280 g (10 oz) brown sugar (about 14 cups)

80 g cocoa powder (about 3 oz)

1 teaspoon powdered baking soda

1 teaspoon sodium chloride

12 tsp. bicarbonate of soda

9 fl oz water (270 ml)

1 teaspoon vanilla extract

sunflower oil, 180 g (6.3 oz)

a single banana

1 Combine the flour, sugar, cocoa powder, baking powder, baking soda, and salt in a mixing dish.

2 Stir in the water, vanilla, and sunflower oil until the batter is smooth and consistent.

3 Cut the banana into thin slices and delicately fold it into the batter.

4 Pour the batter into tiny cupcake molds and bake until done at 180°C (350°F).

Muffins date back to the eighteenth century in England. The name derives from the word moofin, which is a shortened version of the French term moufflet (soft bread).

A clever ruse

If a little wooden toothpick inserted into the muffin comes out dry, it's time to take it out of the oven.

If you'd rather...

When baking muffins, you can use a variety of fruits. Blackberries, blueberries, raspberries, or apples are also wonderful. (Lemon muffins are also shown in this photo.)

Muffins with lemon zest

30 minutes x 10 persons Difficulty

Ingredients

380 g (13.4 oz) flour—approximately 3 12 cup

280 g (10 oz) brown sugar (about 14 cups)

1 teaspoon powdered baking soda

12 tsp. bicarbonate of soda

1 teaspoon sodium chloride

9 fl oz water (270 ml)

1 teaspoon vanilla extract

sunflower oil, 200 g (7 oz)

three lemons

225 g powdered sugar (8 oz)

1 large or 2 small lemons, 75 g (2.6 fl oz) lemon juice

1 Combine the flour, sugar, baking powder, baking soda, and salt in a mixing basin.

2 Combine the water, vanilla, and sunflower oil in a mixing bowl. Mix until the batter is smooth and consistent.

3 Grate the lemon rind and mix it into the batter.

4 Fill mini cupcake molds halfway with batter and bake at 180°C (350°F) until done.

5 To make the lemon glaze, whisk together the powdered sugar and lemon juice until no lumps remain.

6 Finally, drizzle the glaze over the muffins.

There is no mixer.

One distinction between madeleines and muffins is that the latter does not necessitate as much beating of the ingredients. As a result, the dough is less spongy and denser, which is typical of muffins.

* image from the previous page

Chapter Twenty-three

CRUMBLED HAZELNUTS

20 minutes x 5 people x 5 people x 5 people x 5 people x 5 people Difficulty

Ingredients

100 g (3.5 oz) wheat flour (about 34 cup)

100 g (3.5 oz) brown sugar (about 12 cup)

100 g (3.5 oz) hazelnut flour (about 34 cup)

100 g (3.5 oz) margarine (about 1 stick)

1 teaspoon sodium chloride

1 In a mixing basin, combine all of the ingredients.

2 Using a grater, crumble the dough into small pieces and place on a baking dish.

3 Preheat oven to 180°C (350°F) and bake for 8 minutes.

Hazelnut flour is a high-protein and high-fiber food. It can be used to produce various cakes, cookies, and breads.

* On page 203, there is a photo.

Chapter Twenty-four

CRUMBLED APPLES

ten persons

Ingredients

5 apples (Golden Delicious is best)

2 lemons' juice

Cinnamon, 1 teaspoon

100 g (3.5 oz) wheat flour (about 34 cup)

100 g (3.5 oz) almond flour—approximately 12 cup

100 g (3.5 oz) brown sugar (about 12 cup)

100 g (3.5 oz) margarine (about 1 stick)

1 teaspoon sodium chloride

1 Prepare the apples by peeling and dicing them. Toss the fruit in a tray with the lemon juice and cinnamon and set aside.

2 Combine the different flours, sugar, margarine, and salt in a mixing dish.

3 Using a grater, crumble the dough and sprinkle it over the apples.

4 Preheat the oven to 180°C (350°F) and bake the crumble until the top begins to brown.

Crumbles are a traditional English fruit pie prepared with apples, grapes, plums, pears, and other fruits. This dish is thought to have originated during World War II, as a result of food rationing in the United Kingdom during the long struggle.

Sablé with almonds and orange blossoms

20 minutes x 5 people x 5 people x 5 people x 5 people x 5 people Difficulty

Ingredients

100 g (3.5 oz) wheat flour (about 34 cup)

100 g (3.5 oz) brown sugar (about 12 cup)

100 g (3.5 oz) almond flour—approximately 12 cup

100 g (3.5 oz) margarine (about 1 stick)

1 teaspoon sodium chloride

1 teaspoon rind from an orange

1 In a mixing basin, combine all of the ingredients.

2 Place the dough between two sheets of parchment paper and roll it out.

3 Cut out numerous pieces of dough (approximately 4 cm or 1.5 in in diameter) with a cookie cutter and place them on a separate pan.

4 Preheat oven to 180°C (350°F) and bake for 8 minutes.

Shortcrust pastry, also known as sablé, is used to make a variety of cookies as well as sweet and salty tarts including quiches and tartlets. Because of its gritty consistency, it is referred as as sablé (sand) in France.

Chapter Twenty-five

SABLE DE CHOCOLAT

20 minutes x 5 people

Ingredients

70 g (2.5 oz) wheat flour—approximately 12 cup

30 g (1 oz) cocoa powder (about 14 cup)

100 g (3.5 oz) brown sugar (about 12 cup)

100 g (3.5 oz) almond flour—approximately 12 cup

100 g (3.5 oz) margarine (about 1 stick)

1 teaspoon sodium chloride

1 teaspoon vanilla extract

1 In a mixing basin, combine all of the ingredients.

2 Roll out the dough between two pieces of parchment paper using a roller.

3 Cut out numerous pieces of dough (approximately 4 cm or 1.5 in in diameter) with a cookie cutter and place them on a separate pan.

4 Preheat oven to 180°C (350°F) and bake for 8 minutes.

A clever ruse

Allowing the dough to rest before using it is beneficial since it will be much more pliable.

Chapter Twenty-six

CARROT CAKE

Cake with carrots and walnuts

50 minutes x 10 people x 10 people x 10 people x 10 people x 10 people Difficulty

Ingredients

300 g (10.5 oz) whole wheat flour (about 3 cups)

1 teaspoon sodium chloride

270 g (9.5 oz) brown sugar (about 14 cups)

Cinnamon, 1 teaspoon

1 teaspoon bicarbonate of soda

1 teaspoon powdered baking soda

Carrots, 300 g (10.5 oz)—approximately 12 cups

180 g (6.3 oz) sunflower oil (about 34 cup)

200 mL (about 7 fl oz) water

1 teaspoon vanilla extract

130 g (4.5 oz) walnuts—approximately 12 cup

To make the orange icing, combine the following ingredients in a mixing bowl.

300 g (10.5 oz) powdered sugar (about 2 34 cups)

100 g (3.5 fl oz) orange juice (about 12 cup)

1 Combine the flour, salt, sugar, cinnamon, baking soda, and baking powder in a mixing dish.

2 Peel, chop, and grate the carrots finely.

3 In a mixing bowl, combine the oil, water, vanilla, carrots, and nuts. Whisk until the batter is smooth and consistent.

4 Place the batter in a Bundt pan and bake until done at 180°C (350°F).

5 Check the cake with a wooden toothpick to see whether it's done cooking.

6 To prepare the orange icing, whisk together the powdered sugar and orange juice until no lumps remain.

7 Drizzle the icing over the cake and serve.

Chapter Twenty-seven

LOAF CAKE

Loaf cake with blueberries

45 minutes for 6 persons Difficulty

Ingredients

175 g (about 6 oz) flour—around 12 cup

140 g (5 oz) brown sugar (about 58 cup)

12 tblsp. baking powder

12 tsp. bicarbonate of soda

a quarter-teaspoon of salt

5 fl oz water (140 ml)

2 lemons' juice

140 g (5 oz) sunflower oil 1 teaspoon vanilla

100 g (3.5 ounce) blueberries—approximately 12 cup

1 Combine the flour, sugar, baking powder, baking soda, and salt in a mixing basin.

2 Combine the water, lemon juice, vanilla, and sunflower oil in a mixing bowl. Whisk until you have a nice and homogeneous batter.

3 Carefully fold in the blueberries.

4 Pour the batter into a loaf cake pan and bake until done at 180°C (350°F).

If you'd rather...

You can use raspberries instead of blueberries, which will go well with the fresh, acidic flavor of the lemon.

Spheres of chocolate mousse

6 people x 10 minutes x 6 people x 10 minutes x 6 people x 10 minutes Difficulty

Ingredients

100 g (3.5 oz) soy milk—approximately 12 cup

1 bean of vanilla

8 oz. dark chocolate, 225 g

12 cup vegan whipped cream or milk, 125 g (4.5 oz)

If you can't find orange blossom water, use a replacement. 12 teaspoon rind of an orange 1 oz. margarine, 25 g melting chocolate in addition

powdered cocoa

1 Melt the chocolate in a pot with the whipping cream. Bring the water to a boil.

2. Fill an electric blender cup halfway with soy milk. Scrape the vanilla bean's seeds into the soy milk.

3. Slowly drizzle in the boiling cream and emulsify.

4. Mix the orange blossom water and margarine together. Continue mixing until a very fine emulsion forms.

5. Pour the mixture into a dish and lay it in the refrigerator for at least 6 hours.

6. Roll the cubes into spheres after cutting them to the desired size.

7. Drizzle more melted chocolate over the spheres and dust with cocoa powder.

Shots of raisins

30 minutes 6 people Difficulty

Ingredients

200 g (7 oz) raisins (about 1 cup)

50 mL (about 14 cup) rum

a single orange

500 mL (about 2 cups) soy milk

80 g sugar (about 3 oz)

cornstarch, 30 g (1 ounce)

1 Place the raisins in a saucepan, cover with water, and add the shot of rum.

Set aside in tiny glasses after boiling for about 30 minutes over low heat.

2 Peel and grate the orange rind.

3 Bring the milk and sugar to a boil, then add the orange rind.

4 Dissolve the cornstarch in a small amount of water in a bowl. Add to the milk mixture and reheat for 2 minutes over low heat, stirring constantly.

5 To make a couple of well-defined layers, pour the orange crème Anglaise into each small glass, being careful not to overmix with the raisins.

6 Refrigerate for a few hours before serving.

7 Garnish with an orange slice before serving (blood orange).

Soy milk is a vegetable liquid that has fewer sodium and calories than cow's milk and has no lactose, casein (lactic protein), vitamin B12, saturated fats, or cholesterol.

Chapter Twenty-eight

SPONGE CAKE

sponge cake with cherries

50 minutes 6 persons Difficulty

Ingredients

150 g (5.3 oz) wheat flour (about 1 13 cup)

110 g (about 4 oz) sugar—around 12 cup

a quarter teaspoon of

soda bicarbonate

a quarter teaspoon of

powdered sugar

a quarter-teaspoon of salt

cornstarch, 30 g (1 ounce)

100 mL (about 12 cup) sunflower oil

2 lemons' juice

300 g (10.5 oz) pitted and canned cherries (substitute other grain or nut milk, if desired) 140 ml (5 fl oz) oat milk (substitute other grain or nut milk, if desired)

10 g pectin (2 tablespoons)

150 g (about 5 oz) sugar—around 2/3 cup

1 Combine the wheat flour, sugar, baking soda, baking powder, salt, and cornstarch in a mixing dish.

2 Combine the oil, lemon juice, and oat milk in a mixing bowl. Mix everything together until you have a smooth batter.

3 Pour the batter into a form and bake at 170°C (350°F) until cooked through. Keep in a cool, dry place.

4 Next, pit the cherries and use a hand mixer to puree the pulp.

5 Bring the blended cherries to a boil in a pot.

6 Combine the pectin and sugar in a small bowl and slowly drizzle it over the cherries. Wait for it to come to a boil while stirring regularly to keep it from sticking.

7 Spread the cherry marmalade on top of the cake and place it in the refrigerator to cool for 3 hours.

« Oat milk is one of the most delectable vegetable beverages available. It's high in fiber and can aid with cholesterol reduction, gut bacteria, and digestion in general.

« Pectin is a coagulant used in the preparation of marmalade, jams, and jellies. It is derived from vegetable matter in a natural way.

Chapter Twenty-nine

ROSE PETALS AND RASPBERRIES LOAF CAKE

Loaf cake with raspberries and rose petals

30 minutes 6 people Difficulty

Ingredients

1 34 cup wheat flour, 200 g (7 oz)

1 teaspoon sodium chloride

Brown sugar, 120 g (4 oz)

cornstarch, 50 g (about 2 oz)

2 TBS BAKED BAKED BAKED BAKED BAKED B

Sunflower oil, 125 mL (12 cup)

80 mL (3 fl oz) water—approximately 13 cup

2 fl oz rose water, 60 ml

10 raspberries (fresh)

1 Combine the flour, salt, sugar, cornstarch, and baking powder in a mixing dish.

2 Combine the oil, water, and rose water in a mixing bowl. Blend until the batter is smooth and consistent.

3 Pour the batter into a loaf cake pan and gently press the raspberries into the batter.

4 Bake until done at 180°C (350°F).

Sunflower oil is a healthy choice because of its unsaturated fats and vitamin E content, as well as its antioxidant properties. It lowers cholesterol and triglyceride levels in the bloodstream when consumed.

« Raspberries are one of the few fruits that are low in calories (only 32 for every 100 g, or 3.5 oz). Manganese, iron, magnesium, phosphorus, calcium, and potassium are abundant in them.

« Rose water is made by distilling rose petals and is used in a variety of sweets due to its strong flavor and perfume.

Take care...

If you pierce a raspberry with a wooden toothpick to check if the cake is done, you can get confused because the tip will most likely come out moist. In this situation, a second toothpick should be inserted to be sure.

Chapter Thirty

CHOCO COOKIES

12 participants 20 minutes Difficulty

Ingredients

280 g (10 oz) wheat flour (about 2 12 cup)

1 teaspoon sodium chloride

12 tsp. bicarbonate of soda

50 g cocoa powder (about 2 oz)

8 oz margarine (225 g)

220 g (about 8 oz) brown sugar

Dark chocolate, 85 g (3 oz)

1 teaspoon vanilla extract

1 Combine the flour, salt, baking soda, and cocoa powder in a mixing basin.

2 Combine the margarine and sugar in a separate bowl.

3 Toss the flour into the basin with the margarine and stir to combine, being careful not to overwork the mixture or the cookies will be soft.

4 Chop the chocolate into small pieces and combine it with the vanilla in the dough. Mix thoroughly.

5 Shape and place many cookies on a baking sheet, then bake for 10 minutes at 180°C (350°F).

minutes.

Chapter Thirty-one

SACHER

Sachertorte

12 participants 40 minutes Difficulty

Ingredients

2 588 cups wheat flour, 300 g (10.5 oz)

1 teaspoon sodium chloride

brown sugar, 225 g (8 oz)

60 g (2 oz) cocoa powder—approximately 14 cup

1 teaspoon bicarbonate of soda

2 TBS BAKED BAKED BAKED BAKED BAKED B

Water, 250 mL (9 fl oz)

130 mL (about 12 cup) sunflower oil

Apricot

marmalade

Dark chocolate, 200 g (7 oz)

50 g (about 2 oz) sunflower oil 150 g (just over 5 oz) margarine—approximately 1 stick plus 1 tbsp

1 Combine the wheat flour, salt, sugar, cocoa, baking soda, and baking powder in a mixing dish.

2 Whisk together the water and oil until you have a smooth and homogenous batter.

3 Divide the batter into three circular molds (20 cm or 8 in in diameter) and bake until done at 180°C (350°F). Keep in a cool, dry place.

4 Spread marmalade on two of the cake slices and stack all three pieces on top of each other, with the marmalade-free piece on top. Place the cake in the freezer.

5 Melt the chocolate, margarine, and oil together in a double boiler.

Using a hand blender, emulsify the ingredients.

6 Place the cake on a rack and pour the melted chocolate over it completely.

Chapter Thirty-two

CATALONIA CREAM

Difficulty: 6 persons, 10 minutes

Ingredients

agar agar (14 teaspoon)

500 mL (about 2 cups) soy milk

Cinnamon stick, 1

1 lemon's zest

1 orange's zest

80 g sugar (about 3 oz)

corn flour, 20 g (4 teaspoons)

Caramelization sugar

1 Soak the agar agar in the soy milk until it dissolves completely.

2 Combine the cinnamon, lemon and orange rinds, and sugar in a mixing bowl.

Bring the pot of water to a boil.

3 Mix the flour with a little water before adding it to the milk.

4 Heat the mixture in a pot over low heat for a few minutes, stirring regularly.

5 Divide the cream among 6 bowls and chill until ready to use.

6 Before serving, sprinkle it with a little sugar and caramelize it.

Catalan cream is a dessert consisting primarily of cow's milk and eggs. The vegan version is easy to make and tastes just as good. Soy milk and agar agar can be used in place of those items. This final ingredient contributes to the dessert's firm and creamy texture.

Flapjacks

12 participants 15 minutes Difficulty

Ingredients

margarine, 200 g (7 oz)

150 mL (5 fl oz) maple syrup (about 58 cup)

1 12 cup oats (350 g)

1 Melt the margarine in a double boiler and combine it with the maple syrup and oats.

2 Combine the ingredients in a baking dish.

3 Bake at 150°C (300°F) for about 15 minutes, or until the edges are nicely browned.

4 Refrigerate it for 3 hours before cutting it into rectangles and serving.

Flapjacks are a type of miniature cereal bar that originated in England. They're normally made with oats, but you may add any nuts, raisins, dried apricots, etc. They're great for breakfast or a quick snack for kids.

Chapter Thirty-three

FLAPJACKS

12 participants 15 minutes Difficulty

Ingredients

margarine, 200 g (7 oz)

100 mL (3.5 fl oz) maple syrup (about 12 cup)

1 12 cup oats (350 g)

To make the icing:

70 g (2 12 oz) margarine (about 12 stick or 5 tablespoons)

powdered sugar, 200 g (7 oz)

1 teaspoon vanilla extract

1 Melt the margarine in a double boiler and combine it with the maple syrup and oats.

2 After that, transfer the mixture to a baking dish.

3 Bake at 150°C (300°F) for about 15 minutes, or until the edges are nicely browned. Refrigerate any leftovers.

4 In a mixing dish, combine the margarine, sugar, and vanilla extract.

5 Finally, spread the mixture over the flapjacks and cut rectangles out of them.

Chapter Thirty-four

CAKE WITH PLUM AND PISTACHIO

30 minutes 12 people Difficulty

Ingredients

320 g (11 oz) wheat flour—approximately 3 cups

1 teaspoon sodium chloride

270 g sugar (8 oz)

2 TBS BAKED BAKED BAKED BAKED BAKED B

Cinnamon, 1 teaspoon

sunflower oil, 180 mL (34 cup)

Soy milk, 250 mL (1 cup)

120 g (4 oz) plums (about 2 large plums)

50 g (2 oz) hazelnuts—approximately 14 cup

50 g (2 oz) almonds—approximately 14 cup

1 Combine the flour, salt, sugar, baking powder, and cinnamon in a mixing basin.

2 Combine the oil and milk in a mixing bowl. Blend until the batter is smooth and consistent.

3 Toss in the plums, hazelnuts, and almonds.

4 Pour the batter into a rectangular pan, sprinkle with sugar, and bake until done at 180°C (350°F).

Chapter Thirty-five

CAKE WITH A SPONGE TEXTURE

6 participants 25 minutes Difficulty

Ingredients

1 34 cup wheat flour, 200 g (7 oz)

a quarter-teaspoon of salt

1 teaspoon bicarbonate of soda

1 teaspoon powdered baking soda

Cinnamon, 1 teaspoon

agave syrup, 80 mL (13 cup)

sunflower oil, 90 mL (6 tbsp)

110 mL (12 cup) rice milk—other grain or nut milk can be used instead 1 Combine the flour, salt, baking soda, baking powder, and cinnamon in a mixing basin.

2 Combine the syrup, oil, and rice milk in a mixing bowl. Mix until the batter is smooth and consistent.

3 Pour the batter into a small baking pan and bake until done at 150°C (300°F).

« Agave syrup is a sweet vegetable juice made from a cactus species found in the tropical Americas and the Caribbean. Because of its high fructose and glucose content, it has double the sweetening power of regular sugar.

« Rice milk is a vegetable drink that is highly suggested for persons who have stomach problems or have a difficult time digesting food.

Chapter Thirty-six

SCONES WITH BLUEBERRIES

6 participants 25 minutes Difficulty

Ingredients

370 g (13 oz) wheat flour—approximately 3 14 cup

Sugar, 130 g (4.5 oz)

1 tablespoon powdered baking soda

a grain of salt

1 stick of margarine, 120 g (4 oz)

12 cup of water, 130 ml

2 lemons, zest

100 g (3.5 ounce) blueberries—approximately 12 cup

1 Combine the flour, sugar, baking powder, and a pinch of salt in a mixing basin.

2 Add the margarine and knead until the mixture is crumbly.

3 Combine the lemon zest and water in a mixing bowl. Continue to knead the dough.

4 Fold the dough into a disk and add the blueberries.

5 Cut the dough into sixths and bake for 20 minutes at 180°C (350°F).

« Scones are delectable classic English cakes made with berries such as raspberries or blueberries.

« The greatest time to buy blueberries is in June and continues until December.

Look for a bright, lustrous skin tone and select the more fragrant berries when shopping.

« Baking powder is used to expand the volume of dough, and it's especially helpful for creating cakes. It is more effective than baking soda because it begins to work at a lower temperature and has no taste.

Chapter Thirty-seven

COCONUT SPHERES

30 minutes (plus 2 minutes for cooling) 6 people

Ingredients

12 CUP COCONUT OLIVE OIL

1 cup coconut grated

almond flour (1 cup)

12 cup agave nectar

a quarter teaspoon of salt

Coconut grated for dredging

1 In a double boiler, melt the coconut oil until it produces a smooth liquid.

2 Combine the cup of grated coconut, flour, syrup, coconut oil, and salt in a mixing bowl and stir until a homogeneous, firm dough forms.

3 Make little balls out of the dough and roll them in grated coconut.

4 Chill them in the refrigerator for a couple of hours before serving.

Coconut oil is a flavorful and fragrant vegetable oil. It contains a lot of lauric acid, which is found in mother's milk. It's a fantastic ingredient for creating soap and other natural and handmade cosmetics, in addition to its culinary purposes.

CPSIA information can be obtained
at www.ICGtesting.com
Printed in the USA
BVHW011405110722
641843BV00010B/423